MEDITERRENEAN DIET

As you can tell, Mediterranean foods differ depending on which country you're in. Nevertheless, these foods are known worldwide and people will travel from near and far just to indulge in their goodness.

Table Of Contents

SNACKS

Pesto Cream Veggie Dip

This dip recipe is good for sharing with friends as a snack, a tiny meal, or as a dip. Using cream cheese makes it low in phosphate and they would also be small in potassium if served with toasted pitta bread, crackers or maize crisps instead of potato crisps.

Ingredients:

- 200 g (7oz) basil pesto
- 100 g (3 and half oz) cream cheese
- 100 g (3 and half oz) sour cream
- 2 parmesan cheese spoons

Method of preparation

1. Place in a bowl pesto, cream cheese, sour cream and Parmesan cheese and stir well.

2. Mix creamy until ready to serve and chill.

Smoked Mackerel Pate

Enjoy this low phosphate paté on toasted bread, melba toast or any other cracker, if you try to lose weight then choose low fat cream cheese.

Ingredients

- 200 g (7 oz) smoked mackerel fillets, skin removed

- 2 spring onions, trimmed and finely sliced

- 1 lemon● 100 g (3 and half oz) cream cheese

- 1 tablespoon creamed horseradish

Method of Preparation

1. Break the pieces of the mackerel and chop it finely.

2. Add the mackerel, cream cheese, spring onions, creamed horseradish and 1 lemon zest in a bowl and blend together.

3. Squeeze in your zested lemon juice and blend until a coarse paste is in place.

4. Season with pepper to taste.

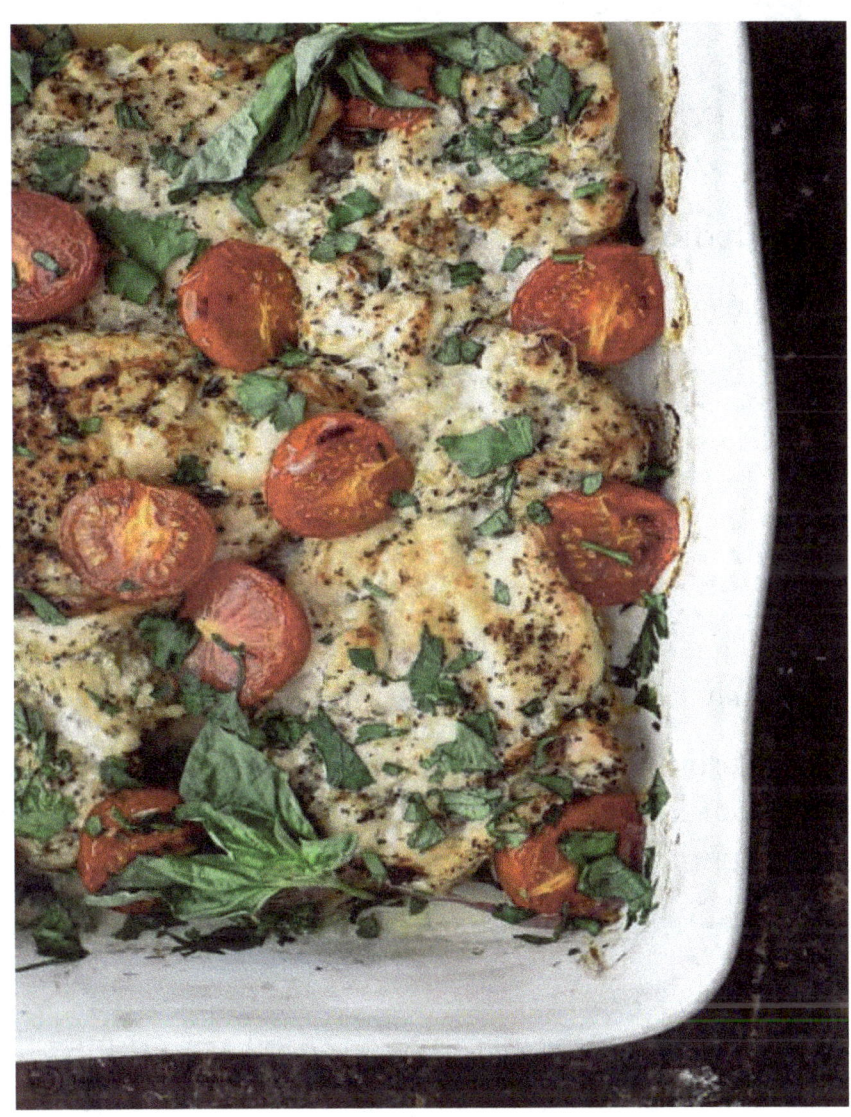

Pancakes

This is really a fast recipe and can be finished with either your selection of sweet or savory ingredients.

Ingredients:

- 1 egg
- 1 cup* of milk
- 1 cup* of flour (any sort)
- Cooking oil or butter* cup= about 200ml

Method of preparation

1. Place in a bowl the egg, milk and flour and whisk to fully mix to create a smooth batter.

2. Add the sunflower oil or butter and a big spoonful of the pancake mixture to heat a frying pan until warm.

3. Fry over medium heat to underneath golden brown.

4. Turn over the pancake and boil for another 1-2 minutes or until golden brown.

5. With the remaining batter, set aside and repeat.

Serving recommendation:

Try with stewed apples or tinned pears, peaches, strawberries or raspberries and serve with single cream (remember tinned fruit is lower in potassium than fresh). Try to serve a delicious pancake with ham, rubbed cheese or tuna.

Plain Scones

This is a staple recipe that works well as a tiny meal, snack or even pudding and is low in potassium as well as phosphate. Making 12 in one go may sound a lot, but they freeze very well–just make sure you use them in a month's time.

Ingredients:

- 225 g (8oz) self-raising flour
- Pinch of salt
- 55 g (2oz) butter
- 25 g (1oz) caster sugar
- 150ml milk
- 1 free-range egg, fried, glazed (alternately using a small amount of milk)

Preparation Technique

1. Heat the oven to a temperature of 220 ° C (200 ° C)/425 ° F / Gas 7. Fat a baking sheet lightly.

2. Salt and flour should be mixed together then add in the butter.

3. To get a smooth dough, add the sugar and then the milk.

Simple Meat Dishes

As part of stew, lamb and pork are very versatile and tasty and can be enjoyed in various forms.

Minted Lamp Chops

While this recipe ideally calls for fresh herbs, with any dried herbs you may have lurking in your cupboard, you can still do this; just decrease the amount by half.

Ingredients:

- 100 g (3 and half oz) breadcrumbs
- 2 tablespoons of fresh mint
- 1 tablespoon of fresh parsley
- 2 lamb chops
- 100 g (3and half oz) flour
- 1 free-range egg, whisked
- 1 tablespoons of vegetable or olive oil

Preparation Technique:

1. Use a blender to blend the breadcrumbs, mint and parsley until well mixed to prepare the lamb chops. Put in a bowl.

2. Coat the chops of the lamb in the flour and dip into the egg until well covered. Pepper season.

3. Heat a medium heat frying pan. Add the oil and put the chops of the lamb in the pan. Cook for 3 minutes.

4. Turn over the chops and boil for another three minutes.

5. Remove the chops and then serve them for three minutes.

Honey Glazed Pork

In this easy to prepare dish, contrasting honey and mustard flavors packs an enormous quantity of flavours. To infuse the flavors into the meat, try marinating the meat overnight.

Ingredients:

- 2 chops of lamb or pork
- 25 g (quarter oz) butter or low fat spread
- 1 tablespoon of honey
- 1tablespoon of mustard
- Black pepper

Preparation Technique:

1. Beat or spread the butter until it is creamy.

2. Blend and season with pepper in the honey and mustard and blend to a soft paste

3. Brush the honey combination about an hour 4 over your chop, cover and stir. Grill the chops 5 minutes each side under a warm grill until cooked and served.

Pan-fried Pork Chop with Creamy leek

Cream is much smaller in potassium and phosphate compared to milk and as such can be enjoyed much more freely on a kidney diet (unless you try to lose weight instead of using half fat cream frache). Using powerful aromas such as leek and garlic can assist flavor foods instead of relying on salt. Serve as rice or couscous with a low potassium starchy food.

Ingredients:

- 2 pork chops
- 1 tablespoon of vegetable or olive oil
- 1 garlic clove, peeled and chopped
- 1/2 leek, washed and sliced
- 2 sprigs of thyme, leaves only
- 50ml milk
- 150ml double cream
- 1 tablespoon of new parsley

Preparation Technique:

1. Heat up to warm a griddle or frying pan. Brush the chop of pork with oil and add six minutes to the pan to boil. Turn over the cut and cook for an additional six minutes or until browned and cooked. When cooked, when pierced with a sharp knife, the juices will run clear. Take off the heat and set aside for three minutes to rest.

2. Heat the oil and butter in a pan for the leeks and sauté the garlic for 3-4 minutes with the leek and thyme leaves to soften.

3. Stir in the milk, cream and parsley, then reduce heat and softly simmer for another 6-8 minutes, occasionally stirring.

4. In the pork chop, spoon the creamed leek sauce and serve.

5. Take the warm tray from the furnace, then mix in the batter rapidly–when it first strikes the warm fat, it should sizzle and bubble a little. Put it back into the oven and bake until the batter is cooked through, well risen and crisp for 40 minutes.

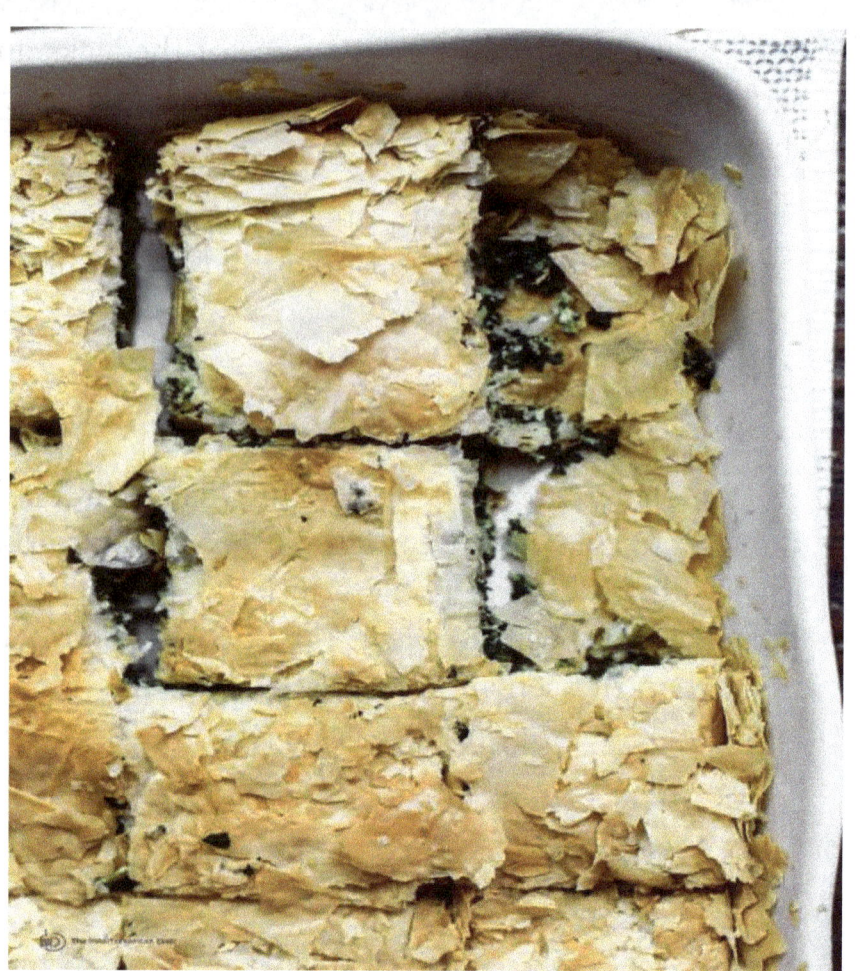

Tomato & cheese tarts

ingredients

2 sheets filo pastry 1 egg white 100g/4oz low-fat soft cheese handful of fresh basil leaves 3 small tomatoes, sliced salt and freshly ground black pepper

Preparation

• Preheat the oven to 200°C/400°F/ Gas mark 6. • Brush the sheets of filo pastry lightly with the egg white, and cut into 16 squares, each measuring about 10cm/4in.

• Layer the squares in twos, in eight patty tins. Spoon the cheese into the pastry cases.

• Season with salt and pepper, and top with the basil leaves.

• Arrange the tomatoes on the tarts, and season again with salt and pepper. Bake for 10–12 minutes until golden. Serve warm.

Succotash

serves 4–6

ingredients

4 tablespoons vegetable oil 500g/1lb 2oz lean smoked bacon rashers, cut into squares 1 large onion, finely sliced 3 garlic cloves, finely chopped 1 red pepper, seeded and chopped 1 green pepper, seeded and chopped 900g/2lb canned red kidney

beans, drained 1.4kg/3lb sweetcorn kernels 3 tomatoes, diced 150g/5oz Parmesan cheese, freshly grated

Preparation

• Heat the oil in a heavy saucepan over a high heat, and sauté the bacon until browned.

• Reduce the heat and add the onion, garlic, peppers, kidney beans and sweetcorn. Pour in 350ml/12fl oz water. Stir well.

• Simmer the succotash over a low heat for 15 minutes, then add the tomatoes. Continue to simmer for a further 20 minutes or until the sauce has reduced.

• Sprinkle the succotash with the cheese, and serve hot.

Szechuan beaten chicken

serves 4

ingredients

2 chicken quarters 1 cucumber, seeded if necessary and cut into matchsticks For the sauce 2 tablespoons light soy sauce 1 teaspoon granulated sugar 1 tablespoon finely chopped spring onions 1 teaspoon red chilli oil 1 /2 teaspoon ground black pepper 1 teaspoon sesame seeds 2 tablespoons smooth peanut butter, creamed with a little sesame oil.

Preparation

• Bring 1 litre/13 /4pt water to a rolling boil in a wok or a large heavy saucepan. Add the chicken quarters, reduce the heat, cover and poach for 30–35 minutes.

• Remove the chicken from the wok or pan, and immerse in a bowl of cold water for at least 1 hour to cool, ready for shredding.

• Remove the chicken pieces from the bowl, drain and pat dry with kitchen paper. Take the meat off the bones. On a flat work surface, pound the chicken with a rolling pin, then tear the meat into shreds using two forks. Mix the chicken with the cucumber, and arrange in a serving dish.

• To serve, mix together all the sauce ingredients until thoroughly combined, and pour over the chicken and cucumber in the serving dish.

Note Sesame oil is very pungent and strong-tasting, so a little of it goes a long way. Use sparingly, adding just a very little at a time, when creaming with the peanut butter, so that it does not overpower the other flavours. You should not need more than a teaspoon or so.

Spinach, feta & pear salad

serves 4

ingredients

2 dessert pears such as Comice, peeled, cored and sliced 4 tablespoons walnut oil 100g/4oz baby spinach leaves 175g/6oz feta cheese, diced 75g/3oz

walnut pieces 1 teaspoon freshly squeezed lemon juice freshly ground black pepper

Preparation

• Toss the pears in a little of the oil.

• In a large salad bowl, combine the spinach, feta cheese and walnut pieces. Gently stir in the pears.

• Whisk together the lemon juice and remaining oil, and season with pepper. Drizzle over the salad.

• Refrigerate, covered, until required.

Grilled artichoke salad

serves 4

ingredients

400g/14oz canned artichoke hearts, drained and halved olive oil for brushing 3 Little Gem lettuces salt and freshly ground black pepper For the dressing 200ml/7fl oz extra virgin olive oil 200ml/7fl ozgrapeseed oil 125ml/4fl oz white wine vinegar pinch of granulated sugar pinch of mustard powder 2 garlic cloves, crushed

Preparation

• Preheat the grill until hot. Season the artichoke hearts with salt and pepper, and brush with olive oil. Grill until charred round the edges.

• To make the dressing, put the oils, vinegar, sugar, mustard powder and garlic into a large screwtop glass jar. Seal the jar and shake well. Season with salt and pepper.

• Toss the lettuces in the dressing with the artichokes, and serve.

Tuscan bean & tuna salad

ingredients

1 small onion, finely chopped 2 x 400g/14oz cans butter beans, drained 2 tomatoes, cut into wedges 175g/6oz canned tuna in oil, drained 2 tablespoons chopped fresh flat-leaf parsley For the dressing 2 tablespoons olive oil 1 tablespoon freshly squeezed lemon juice 2 teaspoons clear honey 1 garlic clove, crushed

Preparation

• Put the onion and butter beans in a bowl, and mix well. Add the tomatoes. Flake the tuna with a fork, and add it to the mixture together with the parsley.

• To make the dressing, mix together the oil, lemon juice, honey and garlic in a screw top glass jar. Seal the jar tightly, and shake until the dressing thickens.

• Pour the dressing over the salad. Toss the ingredients together, and serve straight away

Prawn salad

serves 3–4

ingredients

900g/2lb raw prawns 100g/4oz celery, finely chopped 450g/1lb canned pineapple chunks, drained 75g/3oz raisins 125ml/4fl oz mayonnaise 2 teaspoons curry powder 4 pitta breads 4 leaves of lettuce

Preparation

• Bring a saucepan of water to the boil, add the prawns and cook for 3–5 minutes until the prawns turn pink. Drain and rinse with cold water. Peel and devein the prawns.

• In a bowl, combine the prawns and the remaining ingredients, except the pitta bread and lettuce. Refrigerate for at least 1 hour before serving.

• Serve the prawn salad in the pitta bread with the lettuce leaves.

Classic Caesar salad

serves 6

ingredients

1 small baguette 2 tablespoons olive oil 2 garlic cloves, halved 4 back bacon rashers, trimmed of fat 2 Cos lettuces 10 anchovy fillets in oil, drained and halved lengthways 100g/4oz Parmesan cheese,

freghly grated For the dressing 1 egg yolk 2 garlic cloves, crushed 2 teaspoons Dijon mustard 2 anchovy fillets in oil, drained 2 tablespoons white wine vinegar 1 tablespoon Worcestershire sauce 175ml/6fl oz olive oil salt and freshly ground black pepper

Preparation

• Preheat the oven to 180°C/350°F/Gas mark 4.

• To make the croûtons, cut the baguette into 15 thin slices, and brush both sides of each slice with the oil. Spread the slices out on a baking tray, and bake for 10–5 minutes until golden brown. Leave to cool slightly, then rub each side of each slice of bread with the cut edge of a garlic clove. Cut each slice into small cubes.

• Cook the bacon under a hot grill until crisp. Drain on kitchen paper until cooled, then break into chunky pieces.

• Tear the lettuce leaves into pieces, and put in a large serving bowl with the bacon, anchovies, croûtons and Parmesan.

• For the dressing, put the egg yolks, garlic, mustard, anchovies, vinegar and Worcestershire sauce in a blender or food processor. Season with salt and pepper, and process for 20 seconds or until smooth. With the motor running, gradually add the oil in a thin stream until the dressing is thick and creamy.

• Drizzle the dressing over the salad, and toss very gently until well distributed. Serve immediately

Mussel salad

ingredients

450g/1lb new potatoes 900g/2lb black mussels 175ml/6fl oz dry white wine 1 small onion, sliced 2 sprigs of fresh thyme 2 bay leaves pinch of saffron threads 4 tablespoons sour cream 2 teaspoons chopped fresh parsley salt and ground black pepper

Preparation

• Put the potatoes in a pan of cold, lightly salted water. Bring to the boil, then reduce the heat and simmer for 20 minutes or until tender. Drain and leave to cool.

• Scrub the mussels with a stiff brush and pull out the hairy beards. Discard any broken mussels, or open ones that don't close when tapped on the work surface. Rinse well. Put the wine, onion, thyme, bay leaves and half the mussels in a saucepan with a tight-fitting lid. Cover and cook over a high heat, stirring once, for 4–5 minutes until the mussels start to open. Remove the mussels as they open (discard any that remain closed). Cook the remaining mussels the same way and leave to cool.

• Reserve 125ml/4fl oz of the mussel cooking liquid and strain. While it is still warm, stir in the saffron. Whisk in the sour cream and season well.

• Cut the potatoes into quarters. Remove the mussels and discard the shells. Combine the potatoes and mussels in a bowl, and add the saffron dressing. Sprinkle with the parsley, and serve immediately

Spicy noodle salad

serves 4

ingredients

250g/9oz cooked rice noodles 175g/6oz broccoli, blanched 175g/6oz mangetout, blanched 2 teaspoons sesame oil 2 tablespoons plum sauce 4 tablespoons soy sauce sliced spring onions, to serve chopped fresh red chillies, to serve

Preparation

• In a large bowl, mix the noodles with the broccoli and mangetout, and toss with the sesame oil, plum sauce and soy sauce.

• Sprinkle with the spring onions and chillies, and serve.

Waldorf chicken salad

serves 4

ingredients

500g/1lb 2oz red apples 3 tablespoons freshly squeezed lemon juice 150ml/5fl oz mayonnaise 1 bunch of celery, thinly sliced 4 shallots, sliced 1 garlic clove, crushed 75g/3oz walnuts, chopped

500g/1lb 2oz skinless lean cooked chicken, cubed 1 Cos lettuce salt and ground black pepper

Preparation

• Quarter, core and dice the apples. Put the diced apple in a bowl with the lemon juice and 1 tablespoon of the mayonnaise. Cover with cling film; leave for 40 minutes.

• Add the celery, shallots, garlic and walnuts to the apple, mix then add the remaining mayonnaise and blend thoroughly. Add the chicken and mix well.

• Line a salad bowl with the lettuce leaves. Pile the chicken salad into the centre, season and serve.

Asparagus & potato salad

serves 6

ingredients

450g/1lb small waxy potatoes 125ml/4fl oz extra virgin olive oil 2 shallots, finely chopped) 4 tablespoons white wine vinegar 900g/2lb fresh asparagus tips or young asparagus, trimmed 225g/8oz young spinach leaves, rinsed and drained salt and freshly ground black pepper

Preparation

• Preheat the oven to 220°C/425°F/Gas mark 7.

• Put the potatoes in a roasting tin, drizzle with 1 tablespoon of the oil and season with salt and pepper. Roast for 20–30 minutes until just soft to the centre, then cool.

• Meanwhile, in a small bowl, whisk together some salt, pepper, the shallots, vinegar and the remaining oil. Slice the potatoes thickly, put into a large bowl, pour the dressing over and marinate for 10 minutes.

• Cook the asparagus in lightly salted boiling water for 3–4 minutes. Drain carefully, and put into a bowl of ice-cold water to retain the colour and stop the spears cooking further. Drain again, then add to the potatoes with the spinach. Toss together carefully, and serve

Crab & crispy noodles

ingredients

vegetable oil for deep-frying 50g/2oz Chinese rice noodles 2 cooked crabs 100g/4oz alfalfa sprouts 1 small iceberg lettuce 4 sprigs of fresh coriander, chopped 1 tomato, peeled and diced 4 sprigs of fresh mint, roughly chopped For the dressing 50ml/2fl oz vegetable oil 1 tablespoon sesame oil 1 /2 fresh red chilli, seeded and finely chopped 1 piece preserved stem ginger in syrup, cut into strips, drained, and 2 teaspoons syrup reserved 2 teaspoons light soy sauce juice of 1 /2 lime

Preparation

- To make the dressing, combine the vegetable and sesame oils in a bowl. Add the chilli, ginger and syrup, soy sauce and lime juice.

- Heat the oil in a wok over a high heat. Fry the noodles, one handful at a time, until crisp. Lift out and drain on kitchen paper.

- Flake the white crabmeat into a bowl, and mix well with the alfalfa sprouts. Put the lettuce, coriander, tomato and mint in a serving bowl, pour the dressing over and toss lightly. Place a nest of noodles on top, then add the crabmeat and alfalfa sprouts. Serve.

Simple bean salad

serves 6

ingredients

2 tablespoons olive oil 2 garlic cloves, sliced 2 x 400g/14oz cans flageolet beans, drained and rinsed extra virgin olive oil for drizzling 2 tablespoons basil pesto freshly squeezed lemon juice salt and freshly ground black pepper small handful of fresh basil leaves

Preparation

- Heat the oil in a small heavy pan. Sauté the garlic until golden but not scorched. Stir in the beans, then leave to marinate in the oil for 10–15 minutes.

- When ready to serve, drizzle a little oil over until the beans are generously coated, then add the pesto sauce and lemon juice to taste. Season with salt and pepper, then stir in the basil leaves. Serve straight away.

Tomato & bean salad

serves 10

ingredients

225g/8oz broad beans 225g/8oz French beans, topped and tailed 150ml/5fl oz olive oil 1 garlic clove, crushed 2 tablespoons lemon juice 3 tablespoons chopped fresh basil leaves 100g/4oz mozzarella cheese, diced 700g/11 ?2lb cherry tomatoes, halved salt and freshly ground black pepper

Preparation

• Cook the broad beans in lightly salted boiling water for about 3 minutes, then drain.

• Cook the French beans in lightly salted boiling salted water for 7–10 minutes, then drain.

• Put the oil, garlic and lemon juice in a blender or food processor, and whiz to combine. Stir in the chopped basil and seasoning.

• Mix together the beans, mozzarella and tomatoes. Pour the dressing over and stir to coat completely. Cover and marinate for at least 1 hour before serving.

Crab, melon & cucumber

serves 4

ingredients

2 tablespoons white wine vinegar 150ml/5 floz olive oil salt and ground black pepper 2 tablespoons pickled ginger, chopped 2.5cm/1in piece of fresh root ginger, peeled and grated 225g/8oz fresh cooked white crabmeat, flaked 1 large head chicory, trimmed and leaves separated 1 /2 cucumber, seeded and pared into ribbons 1 charentais melon, peeled, seeded and cut into quarters

Preparation

• Whisk together the vinegar and oil, and season with salt and pepper. In a bowl, toss the crabmeat in half the dressing. Add the pickled ginger and root ginger.

• Arrange a few chicory leaves, cucumber ribbons and a melon quarter on each of four serving plates. Spoon the crabmeat and remaining dressing over the top, and serve.

Black bean & salsa salad

ingredients

425g/15oz canned sweetcorn kernels, drained 425g/15oz canned black beans, drained 200g/7oz celery, chopped 100g/4oz onion, chopped 50g/2oz fresh coriander, chopped 175g/6oz ready-prepared salsa 25ml/1fl oz red wine vinegar 101

Preparation

• Put the sweetcorn, beans, celery, onion and coriander in a large bowl, and mix well. Blend the salsa and vinegar together. Pour over the salad, and toss well.

• Cover and refrigerate for at least 1 hour before serving.

Tofu salad

serves 4

Ingredients

225g/8oz firm tofu, cut into 2cm/3 /4in cubes 100g/4oz mangetout, cut into 3cm/11 /4in lengths 2 small carrots, cut into matchsticks 100g/4oz red cabbage, finely shredded 2 tablespoons chopped peanuts For the marinade 2 teaspoons sweet chilli sauce 1 /2 teaspoon grated fresh root ginger 1 garlic clove, crushed 2 teaspoons light soy sauce 2 tablespoons olive oil

• To make the marinade, put the chilli sauce, ginger, garlic, soy sauce and oil in a screwtop glass jar, and shake well.

• Put the tofu in a medium bowl, pour the marinade over and stir. Cover with cling film and refrigerate for 1 hour.

• Put the mangetout in a small pan, pour boiling water over and leave to stand for 1 minute, then drain and plunge into ice-cold water. Drain well.

• Add the mangetout, carrots and cabbage to the tofu, and toss together lightly. Transfer the salad to a serving bowl, sprinkle with the peanuts and serve immediately.

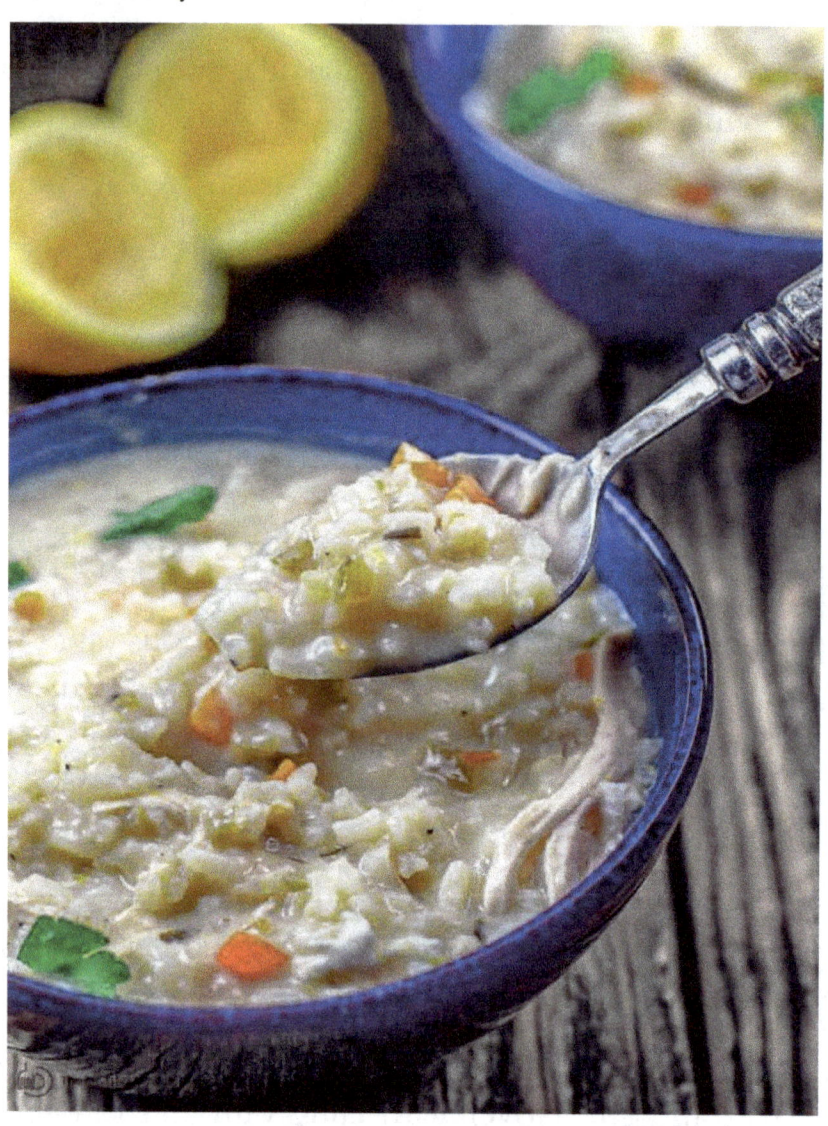

Saffron rice salad

serves 8

ingredients

1 teaspoon saffron threads 6 green cardamom pods 6 cloves 1 cinnamon stick 450g/1lb basmati rice 2 tablespoons olive oil squeeze of lemon juice 50g/2oz flaked almonds, toasted salt and freshly ground black pepper

Preparation

• Put the saffron in a small bowl with 3 tablespoons boiling water, and leave to infuse while the rice is cooking.

• Pour 1 litre/13 /4pt cold water into a pan, season with salt and bring to the boil. Add the spices and rice. Return to the boil, stir with a fork, reduce the heat, cover and simmer for 10 minutes. Stir the rice again, then pour in the saffron liquid without stirring. Cook for a further 5–10 minutes until all of the liquid is absorbed and the rice is tender.

• Put the rice in a bowl and fluff up the grains with a fork. Stir in the oil and lemon juice, and leave to cool. Transfer to a large serving plate, season with salt and pepper, and sprinkle with the almonds.

Borlotti bean salad

serves 4

ingredients

700g/11 /2lb canned cooked borlotti beans, drained 2 garlic cloves 2 tablespoons fresh sage leaves 1 tablespoon red wine vinegar 2 tablespoons French mustard 5 tablespoons extra virgin olive oil 250g/9oz rocket leaves salt and freshly ground black pepper

Preparation

• Put the beans in a saucepan; cover with cold water. Add the garlic and sage leaves. Bring to the boil, and simmer for 5 minutes. Drain, then season with salt and pepper.

• Combine the vinegar and mustard, and season. Slowly whisk in the olive oil.

• Toss the beans with two-thirds of the dressing. Toss the rocket leaves in the remainder of the dressing.

• Divide the dressed leaves between four serving plates. Spoon the beans over the leaves, and serve with the bean juices over the top.

Greek salad

ingredients

4 large beefsteak tomatoes, about 700g/11 /2lb in total 1 large cucumber 2 red onions 1 Cos lettuce

100g/4oz pitted black olives 225g/8oz feta cheese For the dressing 125ml/4fl oz olive oil 50ml/2fl oz lemon juice 3 tablespoons chopped fresh coriander leaves pinch of granulated sugar salt and ground black pepper

Preparation

• Cut the tomatoes into bite-size chunks, discarding the cores. Cut the cucumber in half crossways, then cut a cross in the end of each piece and cut into quarters. Cut the quarters cro

ssways into bite-size pieces. Peel the onions and cut into thin wedges. Shred the lettuce.

• Whisk the dressing ingredients together in a jug. Put all the salad vegetables in a large bowl, add the olives and toss the ingredients together using your hands.

• Pour the dressing over, and toss gently to mix, then crumble over the feta cheese. Serve immediately

Warm pasta & crab

serves 6

ingredients

200g/7oz spaghetti 2 tablespoons olive oil 25g/1oz butter 3 x 200g/7oz canned cooked crabmeat, drained 1 red pepper, cut into thin strips 2 teaspoons finely grated lemon zest 3 tablespoons freshly grated Parmesan cheese 2 tablespoons chopped fresh chives 3 tablespoons chopped fresh flat-leaf parsley salt and ground black pepper

Preparation

• Break the spaghetti in half, and cook in a large pan of lightly salted rapidly boiling water until al dente. Drain.

• Put the spaghetti in a large serving bowl, and toss with the oil and butter. Add the remaining ingredients, and toss to combine.

• Season with salt and pepper, and serve warm.

Tuna & bean salad

serves 4

ingredients

200g/7oz canned tuna in oil 4 spring onions, sliced 2 celery sticks, chopped 400g/14oz canned cannellini beans, drained and rinsed 1 tablespoon drained capers 2 tablespoons chopped fresh flat-leaf parsley For the vinaigrette 2 tablespoons balsamic vinegar 3 tablespoons orange juice juice of 2 limes several dashes of Tabasco sauce 2 garlic cloves, crushed 1 tablespoon caster sugar

Preparation

• To make the vinaigrette, put all the ingredients in a screw-top glass jar, seal tightly and shake well. • To make the salad, put the tuna in a bowl and flake with a fork. Toss in the spring onions and celery, then stir in the beans and capers.

• Pour the vinaigrette over, add the parsley and toss to distribute the dressing evenly. Cover and chill until ready to serve.

Greek cucumber salad

serves 4

ingredients

1 cucumber 1 teaspoon salt 3 tablespoons finely chopped fresh mint 1 garlic clove, crushed 1 teaspoon caster sugar 200ml/7fl oz Greek-style yogurt

Preparation

• Peel the cucumber and cut in half lengthways. Remove the seeds with a teaspoon and discard. Slice the cucumber thinly. Put in a bowl, and sprinkle with the salt. Toss through, and leave for at least 15 minutes.

• Combine the mint, garlic, sugar and yogurt in another bowl.

• Rinse the cucumber in a sieve under cold running water to flush away the salt.

• Drain well and combine with the yogurt mixture. Chill for 15 minutes and serve.

Salad niçoise

ingredients

3 eggs 2 vine-ripened tomatoes 175g/6oz baby green beans, trimmed 125ml/4fl oz olive oil 2 tablespoons white wine vinegar 1 garlic clove, halved 350g/12oz iceberg lettuce heart, cut into 8 wedges 1 red pepper, seeded and thinly sliced 1 cucumber, cut into 5cm/2in lengths 1 celery stick, cut into 5cm/2in lengths 1 /4 large red onion, thinly sliced 350g/12oz canned tuna, drained 12 pitted black olives 2 x 175g/6oz cans anchovy fillets in oil, drained 2 teaspoons baby capers, drained 12 small fresh basil leaves

Preparation

• Put the eggs in a saucepan of cold water. Bring to the boil, then reduce the heat and simmer for 10 minutes. Stir during the first few minutes to centre the yolks. Cool under cold water, then peel and cut into quarters. Meanwhile, score a cross in the base of each tomato, and put in a bowl of boiling water for 10 seconds. Plunge into cold water and peel away from the cross. Cut each tomato into eight sections.

• Cook the beans in a saucepan of boiling water for 2 minutes, rinse under cold water, then drain.

• For the dressing, put the oil and vinegar in a screwtop glass jar, seal tightly and shake to combine.

• Rub the garlic over the bottom and sides of a platter. Arrange the lettuce over the bottom. Layer the egg, tomato, beans, red pepper, cucumber and celery over the lettuce. Scatter the onion and tuna over them, then the olives, anchovies, capers and basil. Drizzle the salad with the dressing, and serve.

Thai noodle salad

serves 4

ingredients

250g/9oz thin instant noodles 450g/1lb cooked large prawns, peeled, deveined and halved lengthways 5 spring onions, sliced 2 tablespoons chopped fresh coriander leaves 1 red pepper, chopped 100g/4oz mangetout, sliced For the dressing 2 tablespoons grated fresh root ginger 2 tablespoons light soy sauce 2 tablespoons sesame oil 75ml/3fl oz red wine vinegar 1 tablespoon sweet chilli sauce 2 garlic cloves (crushed) 75ml/3fl ozkecapmanis

Preparation

• To make the dressing, put the ingredients in a large bowl, and whisk together with a fork.

• Cook the noodles in a large pan of boiling water for 2 minutes, then drain well. Add to the dressing and mix well. Leave to cool.

• Add the prawns and remaining ingredients to the noodles, and toss through gently. Serve at room temperature. salads 106 Couscous & haddock salad serves 2 ingredients 175g/6oz couscous 100g/4oz cooked, flaked smoked haddock 50g/2oz cooked green peas pinch of curry powder 2 spring onions, sliced 1 small egg, hard-boiled and chopped 2 tablespoons olive oil 2 tablespoons freshly squeezed lemon juice salt and freshly ground black pepper

• Cook the couscous according to the packet instructions.

• Mix the couscous with the haddock, peas, curry powder, spring onions and chopped egg.

• Toss with the olive oil and lemon juice, and season with plenty of salt and pepper.

Thai beef salad

ingredients

vegetable oil for frying 450g/1lb lean rump steak 3 tablespoons freshly squeezed lime juice 3 tablespoons Thai fish sauce 1 tablespoon granulated sugar 4 shallots, thinly sliced 2 garlic cloves, crushed 2 fresh red chillies, seeded and finely sliced 6–8 lettuce leaves 1 tablespoon chopped fresh coriander leaves 1 tablespoon chopped fresh chives 1 /2 cucumber, peeled and cut into slices 5mm/1 /4in thick 2 tomatoes, cut into eighths• Preheat the oven to 240°C/ 450°F/Gas mark 8.

Preparation

• Heat a little oil in a flameproof dish until it is very hot. Add the meat and brown it quickly over a fierce heat. Transfer to the oven, and roast for 10–15 minutes.

• Leave to rest for at least 5 minutes, then slice thinly.

• Mix together the lime juice, fish sauce and sugar, stirring until the sugar has dissolved. Add the shallots, garlic and chillies.

• Make a bed of lettuce on a serving dish, and pile the beef in the centre. Spoon the dressing over and scatter with coriander and chives. Arrange the cucumber and tomato wedges around the edge of the salad, and serve.

Curly endive salad

serves 4

ingredients

1 /2 curly endive 1 /2 small onion, very thinly sliced grated zest and juice of 1 /2 lemon 1 teaspoon clear honey 2 teaspoons walnut oil salt and freshly ground black pepper

Preparation

• Tear the curly endive into neat pieces, and put in a large salad bowl. Scatter the onion over.

• Whisk together the lemon zest, juice, honey, oil and 2 teaspoons water. Season with salt and pepper, and whisk again.

• Drizzle the dressing over the endive, and serve.

Chinese prawn salad

serves 6

ingredients

175g/6oz beansprouts 1 small red pepper, chopped
100g/4oz peeled and deveined cooked prawns 2
teaspoons light soy sauce 2 teaspoons white wine
vinegar 1 /2 teaspoon granulated sugar 2
tablespoons sesame oil salt and freshly ground black
pepper 6 large lettuce leaves 1 spring onion,
chopped

Preparation

• Put the beansprouts in a bowl with the pepper and
prawns.

• Mix together the remaining ingredients except the
lettuce and spring onion, and pour over the prawn
mixture. Toss well.

• Put a lettuce leaf in the bottom of each of six
individual bowls. Spoon some prawn mixture on to
each lettuce leaf, and scatter the spring onion over
the top. Serve.

Smoked mackerel salad

serves 6

ingredients

450g/1lb new potatoes, halved lengthways 4
tablespoons extra virgin olive oil 3 smoked

mackerel fillets, skinned and broken into strips 250g/9oz cherry tomatoes, halved 1 /2 cucumber, seeded and diced 75g/3oz watercress 2 teaspoons horseradish sauce 2 tablespoons white wine vinegar salt and freshly ground black pepper

Preparation

• Put the potatoes in a pan of cold water, cover and bring to the boil. Cook for 10 minutes or until tender. Drain well, tip back into the pan and add 1 tablespoon of the oil. Season well with salt and pepper. Cover the pan and shake well to mix. Spoon the potatoes into a large bowl.

• Add the mackerel, tomatoes and cucumber, and top with the watercress and a pinch of salt and pepper.

• Mix together the horseradish, remaining oil and the vinegar in a bowl, and season well with salt and pepper. • Pour the dressing over the salad. Toss gently, and serve.

Tomato & spring onion salad

ingredients

8 ripe tomatoes 3 spring onions, finely sliced 1 tablespoon olive oil 1 tablespoon white wine vinegar 1 /2 teaspoon granulated sugar salt and freshly ground black pepper

Preparation

• Put the tomatoes in a bowl of just- boiled water for 30 seconds. Remove with a slotted spoon, then peel off and discard the skin. Cut the flesh into wedges.

• Put the tomatoes in a dish, and sprinkle with the spring onions.

• Whisk together the remaining ingredients and drizzle over the top. Leave to stand for 30 minutes before serving.

Pear & grape salad

serves 4

ingredients

2 teaspoons skimmed milk 225g/8oz low-fat cottage cheese, whipped 1 teaspoon granulated sugar 2 large pears, halved, peeled and cored 8 iceberg lettuce leaves 20 seedless white grapes, halved

Preparation

• Mix the milk with the cottage cheese and sugar, and blend until of a spreading consistency.

• Put the pear halves on the lettuce leaves, cut side down, and frost generously with the cottage cheese.

• Press the grapes, cut side down, into the cottage cheese.

• Chill the salad for at least 20 minutes before serving.

Baked seafood salad

serves 6

ingredients

1 small green pepper, seeded and chopped 1 small onion, chopped 225g/8oz celery, chopped 450g/1lb cooked crabmeat 450g/1lb small cooked scallops 225g/8oz low-fat sour cream 1 teaspoon salt 1 teaspoon Worcestershire sauce 225g/8oz coarse breadcrumbs 25g/1oz margarine

Preparation

• Preheat the oven to 180°C/ 350°F/Gas mark 4.

• Mix all the ingredients except the breadcrumbs and margarine in a casserole dish. Sprinkle the breadcrumbs over the top, and dot with the margarine. Bake for 30 minutes, and serve warm.

Brown rice & chicken salad

serves 8

ingredients

450g/1lb brown rice 450g/1lb lean skinless cooked chicken, diced 12 spring onions, sliced 2 celery sticks, chopped 2 green peppers, seeded and chopped 100g/4oz black olives, pitted and halved 50g/2oz pimiento, minced 100g/4oz cherry tomatoes, halved 100g/4oz fresh flat-leaf parsley, chopped 100g/4oz radishes, sliced 50ml/2fl oz olive oil 50ml/2fl oz white wine vinegar

Preparation

• In a covered saucepan, cook the rice in 450ml/3 /4pt water over a medium heat for about 25 minutes or until the liquid is absorbed and the rice is fluffy. Remove from the heat and leave to cool.

• Add all the remaining ingredients and toss well.

Nutty rice salad

ingredients

175g/6oz long-grain rice 50g/2oz frozen peas 50g/2oz raisins 50g/2oz toasted flaked almonds 2 tablespoons sunflower oil 1 tablespoon white wine vinegar salt and freshly ground black pepper

Preparation

• In a covered saucepan, cook the rice in 175ml/6fl oz water over a medium-high heat for about 20 minutes. Add the peas and cook for a further 5 minutes. Drain, rinse with cold water, and drain again. Empty into a salad bowl.

• Add the raisins, almonds, oil and vinegar. Season with salt and pepper. Toss well and serve.

Rocket salad

serves 4

ingredients

1 slice white bread, cubed 1 garlic clove, quartered 1 tablespoon low-fat spread 100g/4oz rocket leaves 1 sprig of fresh coriander, leaves picked 1 sprig of fresh flat leaf parsley, leaves picked 1 red onion, sliced 1 tablespoon tarragon vinegar salt and freshly ground black pepper

Preparation

• Put the bread, garlic and low-fat spread in a small heavy frying pan over a gentle heat, and toss until golden. Remove from the heat, discard the garlic and drain the croûtons on kitchen paper. • Put the rocket, coriander and parsley in a small salad bowl. Scatter the onion and croûtons over the top of the greens. Sprinkle with the vinegar, and season well with salt and pepper. Serve.

Beetroot & orange salad

serves 4

ingredients

1 Little Gem lettuce, leaves separated 2 oranges 2 large cooked beetroot, diced 1 tablespoon orange juice 1 teaspoon balsamic vinegar salt and freshly ground black pepper

Preparation

- Divide the lettuce leaves evenly among four small serving plates.

- Holding the oranges over a bowl, remove all the pith and zest. Cut the flesh into segments. Squeeze any juice from the membranes into the bowl, then discard them.

- Pile the beetroot in the centre of the lettuce leaves with the orange segments surrounding them. • Add the orange juice to the bowl with the vinegar. Season with salt and pepper. Spoon the dressing over the beetroot, and serve.

Hot potato & bean salad

serves 4

ingredients

450g/1lb potatoes, scrubbed and diced 100g/4oz French beans, topped and tailed, cut into short lengths 75ml/3fl oz low-fat crème fraîche 2 teaspoons chopped fresh mint salt and freshly ground black pepper

Preparation

- Cook the potatoes in lightly salted boiling water for 5 minutes.

- Add the beans to the potatoes, and cook for a further 5–10 minutes until the potatoes are tender. Drain and return to the pan.

- Add the crème fraîche and mint, and season with salt and pepper. Toss gently, and serve warm.

Fresh salad with raspberry vinaigrette

ingredients

1 bunch watercress, torn 2 heads Bibb lettuce, torn into bite-size pieces 450g/1lb mushrooms, sliced 425g/15oz canned artichoke hearts, drained 1 bunch white radishes, sliced 225g/8oz fresh raspberries For the vinaigrette 125ml/4fl oz raspberry vinegar 1 /2 teaspoon salt 225g/8oz olive oil 1 /2 teaspoon Dijon mustard 1 /2 teaspoon freshly ground black pepper

Preparation

• Put the watercress, lettuce, mushrooms, artichoke hearts and radishes in a large bowl.

• Shake the vinaigrette ingredients together in a screwtop glass jar, and drizzle over the salad. Toss well. Serve with the raspberries scattered over the top

Beetroot & chive salad

serves 4

ingredients

4 cooked beetroot, chopped 2 tablespoons low-fat cr?mefra?che 1 tablespoon snipped fresh chives salt and freshly ground black pepper

Preparation

• Put the beetroot in a bowl. Add the crème fraîche, and season with salt and pepper.

- Sprinkle over the chives, toss and serve immediately.

Mustard carrot salad

serves 4

ingredients

450g/1lb carrots, coarsely grated 25g/1oz low-fat spread 1 tablespoon mustard seeds 1 tablespoon freshly squeezed lemon juice salt and freshly ground black pepper

Preparation

- Put the carrots in a salad bowl, and season with salt and pepper.

- Melt the low-fat spread in a frying pan over a medium heat, and add the mustard seeds.

- When they start to pop, add the lemon juice, stir and pour over the salad. Toss well and serve straight away, while still warm.

Banana & pecan salad

serves 6

ingredients

50g/2oz finely chopped lean back bacon 50g/2oz pecan nuts, chopped 200g/7oz banana, sliced 300g/11oz celery, sliced 1 /2 lime, thinly sliced

250g/9oz low-fat Greek-style yogurt 6 lettuce leaves

Preparation

• Grill the bacon until crisp, then cut into small pieces.

• Mix together the bacon, pecan nuts, banana, celery, lime and yogurt in a bowl.

• Put a lettuce leaf on the bottom of each of six individual bowls, and divide the mixture between each bowl.

Turnip salad

ingredients

350g/12oz turnips 2 spring onions, white part only, chopped 1 tablespoon caster sugar pinch of salt 2 tablespoons horseradish cream 2 teaspoons caraway seeds

Preparation

• Peel, slice and shred the turnips. Add the spring onions, sugar and salt, then rub together with your hands to soften the turnip.

• Fold in the horseradish cream and caraway seeds, and serve.

Cranberry cream salad

serves 6

ingredients

75g/3oz cherry elatine 225ml/8fl oz hot water 450g/1lb cranberry sauce 100g/4oz celery, diced 50g/2oz raisins 225g/8oz low-fat sour cream

Preparation

• Dissolve the gelatine in the hot water, and chill until slightly thickened. Fold the cranberry sauce into the gelatine, and add the celery and raisins.

• Fold in the sour cream, and pour the mixture into a mould. Chill until firm, then turn out and serve.

Basque tomatoes

serves 8

ingredients

8 firm ripe tomatoes 100g/4oz fresh flat-leaf parsley, chopped 1 garlic clove, crushed 1 teaspoon salt 1 teaspoon granulated sugar 1 /4 teaspoon coarse-ground black pepper 100g/4oz black olives 50ml/2fl oz olive oil 2 tablespoons tarragon vinegar 1 teaspoon Dijon mustard

Preparation

• Slice the tomatoes, spread them in a shallow dish and sprinkle with the parsley.

• Combine the remaining ingredients in a bowl, mix well and pour over the tomatoes. Cover with cling film, and refrigerate for at least 2 hours before serving.

Spinach & bacon salad

serves 4

ingredients

1 slice white bread, crusts removed 1 tablespoon low-fat spread 3 rashers rindless streaky back bacon, diced 175g/6oz spinach leaves, torn into pieces 1 small onion, thinly sliced and separated into rings 1 tablespoon olive oil 2 teaspoons red wine vinegar 1 teaspoon Worcestershire sauce freshly ground black pepper

Preparation

• Spread the bread with the low-fat spread on both sides, and cut into small dice.

• Sauté the bread cubes in a frying pan until golden. Remove from the pan, and drain on kitchen paper.

• Wipe out the pan, add the bacon and fry until crisp. Remove from the pan. Drain on kitchen paper.

• Put the spinach in a salad bowl with the onion. Whisk together the oil, vinegar, Worcestershire sauce and some pepper.

• Drizzle the dressing over the salad, and top with the croûtons.

Bamboo shoot salad

. ingredients

400g/14oz canned whole bamboo shoots 25g/1oz long-grain rice 2 tablespoons chopped shallots 1 tablespoon chopped garlic 3 tablespoons chopped spring onion 2 tablespoons Thai fish sauce 2 tablespoons lime juice 1 teaspoon granulated sugar 1/2 teaspoon dried red chilli flakes 20 small fresh mint leaves 1 tablespoon sesame seeds, toasted 117

Preparation

• Rinse and drain the bamboo shoots, then slice and set aside in a serving bowl.

• Dry-roast the rice in a heavy frying pan until it is golden brown. Remove and grind to fine crumbs using a mortar and pestle.

• Tip the ground rice into a bowl. Add the shallots, garlic, spring onions, fish sauce, lime juice, sugar, chilli flakes and half of the mint leaves. Mix thoroughly.

• Pour over the bamboo shoots, and toss together. Serve the salad sprinkled with the sesame seeds and the remaining mint leaves

Beansprout & pepper salad

serves 4

ingredients

175g/6oz beansprouts 1 red pepper, seeded and cut into thin rings 1 green pepper, seeded and cut into thin rings 1 onion, thinly sliced and separated into rings For the dressing 2 tablespoons light soy sauce

1 tablespoon sherry salt and freshly ground black pepper

Preparation

• To make the dressing, put all the ingredients in a screwtop glass jar, add 2 tablespoons water, seal tightly and shake well. • Mix together the beansprouts, peppers and onion in a large salad bowl. Pour over the dressing, toss gently and serve.

Fruity pasta & prawn salad

serves 6

ingredients

175g/6oz pasta shells 225g/8oz frozen prawns, thawed and drained 1 large cantaloupe melon 2 tablespoons olive oil 1 tablespoon tarragon vinegar 2 tablespoons snipped fresh chives 200g/7oz Chinese leaves, shredded

Preparation

• Cook the pasta in lightly salted boiling water until al dente. Drain well and allow to cool. • Peel the prawns, and discard the shells.

• Halve the melon, and remove the seeds with a teaspoon. Scoop the flesh into balls with a melon baller, and mix with the prawns and pasta.

• Whisk the oil, vinegar and chives together. Pour over the prawn mixture, and toss to coat. Cover and chill for at least 30 minutes.

• Use the Chinese leaves to line a shallow bowl. Pile the prawn mixture onto the leaves, and serve.

Cucumber salad

serves 6

ingredients

3 large cucumbers, peeled and thinly sliced 1 large red onion, sliced and separated into rings 125ml/4fl oz white vinegar 3 tablespoons granulated sugar 1 teaspoon salt 1 /4 teaspoon pepper 1 /4 teaspoon ground ginger 1 tablespoon snipped fresh chives

Preparation

• Layer the cucumbers in a bowl. Add the onion.

• Put the vinegar, sugar, salt, pepper, ginger and chives in a screwtop glass jar. Seal tightly and shake well to combine.

• Pour the dressing over the cucumbers, and refrigerate for at least 1 hour before serving

Hot bulgur salad

ingredients

100g/4oz bulgur wheat 1 teaspoon salt 2 tablespoons olive oil 2 tablespoons freshly squeezed lemon juice 1 garlic clove, finely chopped 2 tablespoons chopped fresh flat-leaf parsley 1 tablespoon chopped fresh mint 1 teaspoon chopped fresh coriander leaves 3 ripe tomatoes, chopped 5cm/2in piece of cucumber, chopped 1 green pepper, seeded and chopped 4 black olives, pitted and halved

• Put the bulgur in a pan. Add 250ml/9fl oz boiling water and sprinkle with the salt. Stir and leave to stand for 20 minutes until the bulgur has absorbed all the water.

• Add the oil, lemon juice, garlic, herbs, tomatoes, cucumber and green pepper. Toss over a gentle heat for 1 minute.

• Pile the salad onto individual serving plates, and garnish with the olives before serving.

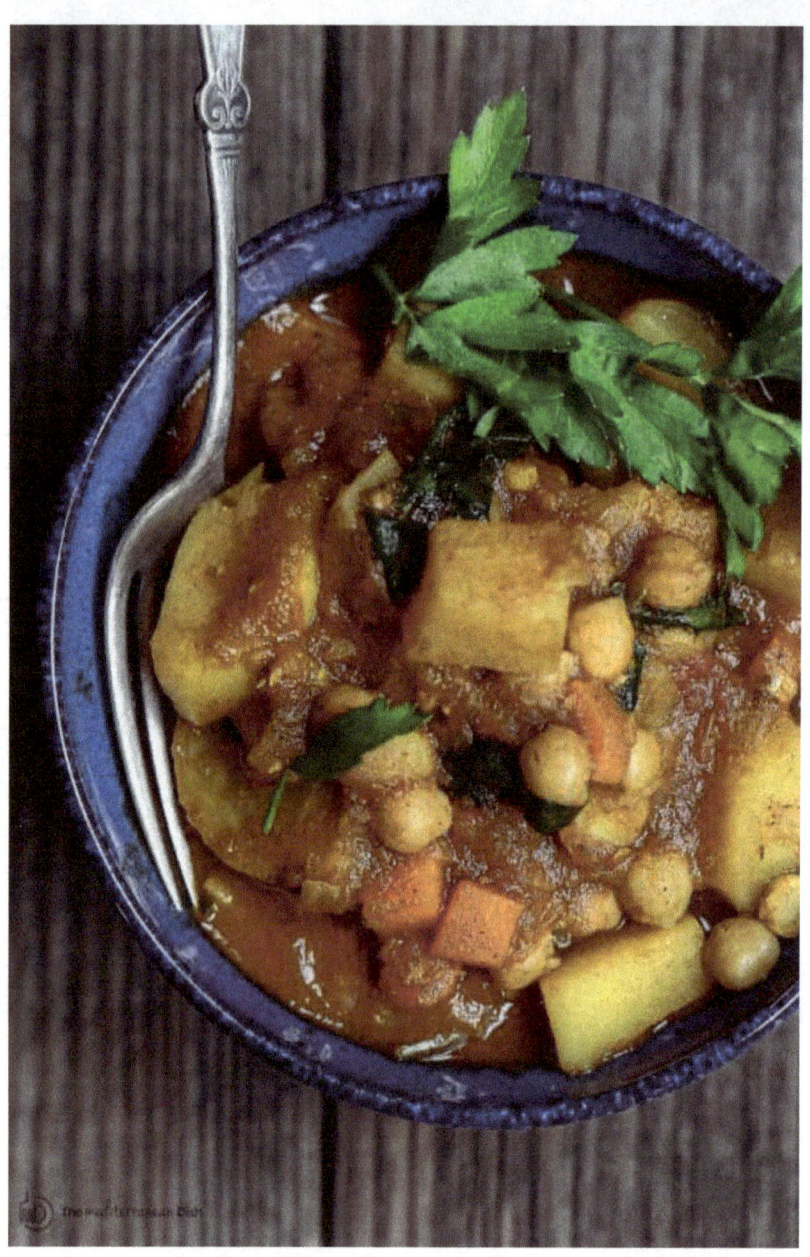

Banana & chicory salad

serves 4

ingredients

2 bananas, thickly sliced grated zest and juice of 1 lemon 2 heads chicory 1 tablespoon sunflower oil 1 teaspoon granulated sugar 1 tablespoon chopped fresh coriander leaves 1 tablespoon desiccated coconut, toasted salt and freshly ground black pepper

Preparation

• Toss the bananas in a little of the lemon juice to prevent browning.

• Cut a cone-shaped core out of the base of each chicory head, then separate into leaves. Arrange the leaves on a serving plate, and pile the bananas in the centre.

• Whisk together the remaining lemon juice, zest, oil and sugar. Season with salt and pepper, and whisk again.

• Pour the dressing over the salad. Sprinkle with the coriander and coconut. Serve straight away. serves 4

Orange & chicory salad

serves 4

ingredients

1 head radicchio 1 head chicory 2 oranges 75g/3oz raspberries 1 tablespoon raspberry vinegar 1 tablespoon freshly squeezed orange juice freshly ground black pepper

Preparation

• Separate the radicchio into leaves, and tear into small pieces. Cut a cone-shaped core out of the base of the chicory, cut the head into chunks, then separate the layers.

• Cut off all the zest and pith from the oranges. Cut the fruit into thin rounds, then slice each round into quarters. Mix together with the salad leaves, and spoon on to four individual serving plates.

• Scatter over the raspberries, and add a good grinding of pepper. Whisk together the vinegar and orange juice, and drizzle over the salad just before serving.

Broccoli salad

serves 4

ingredients

900g/2lb fresh broccoli 225g/8oz fresh mushrooms, sliced 100g/4oz low-fat sour cream 100g/4oz low-fat mayonnaise 1 teaspoon granulated sugar pinch of freshly ground black pepper 1 teaspoon grated onion 1 garlic clove, crushed 225g/8oz canned water chestnuts, drained and sliced

Preparation

• Cut off and discard the tough ends of the broccoli stalks. Break the florets into small clusters, and steam for about 10 minutes until al dente. Refresh in cold water and Drain.

• Mix together the mushrooms, sour cream, mayonnaise, sugar, pepper, onion and garlic in a small bowl.

• In a large salad bowl, combine the broccoli and water chestnuts. Add the creamed mixture, and toss gently. Cover with cling film, and refrigerate for at least 4 hours before serving.

Crispy cheese balls

serves 6

ingredients

250ml/8fl oz milk 250g/9oz plain flour 75g/3oz butter 250g/9oz Cheddar cheese, grated 1 teaspoon cayenne pepper 3 eggs, beaten salt vegetable oil for deep-frying

Preparation

• Warm the milk in a large heavy saucepan over a medium heat, stirring constantly while gradually adding the flour.

• Add the butter and, once the mixture has thickened, remove from the heat and mix in the cheese.

- Add salt to taste, the cayenne and the beaten eggs.

- Allow the mixture to cool. It should now be thick enough to shape into about 24 balls.

- Heat the oil in a deep heavy saucepan until very hot. Deep-fry the balls in batches of about six until they are golden brown.

- Remove from the pan with a slotted spoon, drain on kitchen paper and serve immediately.

Egg salad

serves 4

ingredients

8 eggs, hard-boiled and chopped 50g/2oz butter 4 tablespoons chopped celery 2 tablespoons small capers, rinsed and drained 2 teaspoons grain mustard 1 teaspoon chopped fresh tarragon salt and freshly ground black pepper

Preparation

- In a large bowl, mix all the ingredients thoroughly, seasoning to taste with salt and pepper.

• Serve on a bed of crisp lettuce.

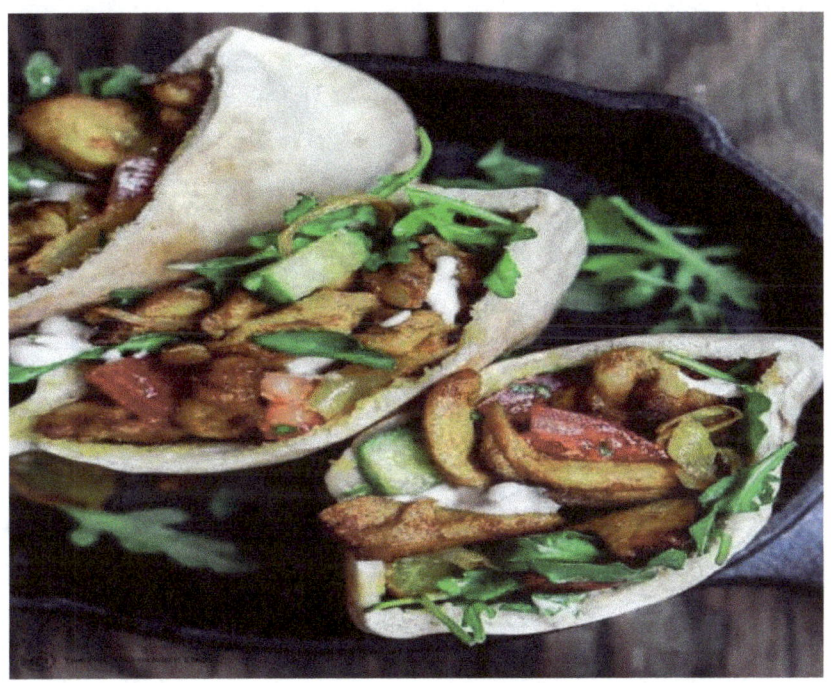

Quail's egg & tomato salad

ingredients

50g/2oz pine nuts 125ml/4fl oz olive oil 24 cherry tomatoes 24 quail's eggs, hard-boiled and chopped 1 /2 teaspoon salt 1 /2 teaspoon granulated sugar 2 tablespoons red wine vinegar

Preparation

• In a frying pan over a medium heat, fry the pine nuts in a teaspoon of the oil until golden brown, taking care not to scorch.

• Put the tomatoes and quail's eggs in a serving bowl. Sprinkle the pine nuts over the top.

• Blend the remaining olive oil, salt, sugar and red wine vinegar together in a screw-top glass jar until thoroughly mixed.

• Pour the dressing over the eggs. Let stand for 10 minutes to allow the flavours to infuse before serving.

Eggs with spinach

serves 2

ingredients

450g/1lb fresh spinach 25g/1oz butter 1 small onion, finely chopped pinch of ground nutmeg 4 eggs salt and freshly ground black pepper

Preparation

- Cook the spinach for 1–2 minutes in boiling water until the leaves have just wilted, then drain and squeeze out the excess water.

- In a heavy frying pan, melt the butter and sweat the onion for 5 minutes until soft.

- Add the spinach and cook for a further 5 minutes, stirring frequently. Season with a pinch of nutmeg and salt and pepper.

- Make four holes in the spinach, and break an egg into each space.

- Cover the pan and cook for 5 minutes until the egg whites are cooked through.

- Serve with bread. serves 4

Feta cheese & capers

serves 6

ingredients

1 /2 teaspoon mixed peppercorns 8 coriander seeds 350g/12oz feta cheese, cubed 2 garlic cloves, thinly sliced 1 bay leaf 1 tablespoon capers, rinsed and drained 1 sprig of fresh oregano or thyme olive oil to cover 16 black olives hot toast

Preparation

- Using a mortar and pestle, lightly crush the peppercorns and coriander seeds.

- In a screwtop glass jar, layer the feta cheese, garlic, bay leaf, ground peppercorns and coriander seeds, capers and a fresh sprig of thyme or oregano.

- Pour in enough oil to cover the cheese, and marinate for 2 weeks in the refrigerator.

- Serve the feta cheese on hot toast together with the black olives and a drizzling of oil.

Camembert with garlic

serves 4

ingredients

1 whole Camembert housed in a wooden box 4 garlic cloves, thickly sliced 4 thick slices brown bread, crusts removed 4 teaspoons cranberry sauce fresh watercress, to garnish

Preparation

- Preheat the oven to 200°C/ 400°F/Gas mark 6.

- Remove the cheese from its packaging, retaining the wooden box. Quarter the cheese, then put back in the wooden box, excluding any paper.

- Slip the garlic slices in the gaps between the quarters. Bake in the oven for 8–10 minutes until the cheese is very soft and warm.

- Serve on a bed of lightly toasted brown bread accompanied by the cranberry sauce and garnished with watercress.

Fried mozzarella

ingredients

4 eggs 15g/1 /2oz plain flour, seasoned with salt and freshly ground black pepper 15g/1 /2oz dried white breadcrumbs 600g/11 /4lb mozzarella cheese sunflower oil for deep-frying

Preparation

• Beat the eggs in a bowl. Spread some seasoned flour on one plate and some breadcrumbs on another.

• Slice the mozzarella into 5mm/1 /2in pieces. Dredge the slices with the flour first, then dip into the beaten egg, then into the breadcrumbs. Dip again into the egg and again into the breadcrumbs to coat well.

• Pour the sunflower oil into a deep heavy frying pan so that it is at least 2.5cm/1in in depth. Heat until a piece of bread dropped into the oil sizzles immediately.

• Fry the coated cheese in the oil until golden. Remove with a spatula, drain on kitchen paper and serve hot.

Parmesan balls

serves 6

ingredients

vegetable oil for deep-frying 175g/6oz Parmesan cheese, freshly grated 2 egg whites, stiffly beaten 1 /2 teaspoon cayenne pepper

Preparation

• Heat the oil in a large heavy pan until very hot.

• Mix the Parmesan with the egg whites and cayenne, keeping aside a small quantity of cheese for dusting the balls.

• Using the remaining cheese to dust your hands, form the mixture into 12 small balls.

• Deep-fry the balls in two batches until golden brown. Drain and serve immediately.

Ricotta cheese &courgette rolls

serves 2

ingredients

2 large courgettes, cut lengthways into 1cm/1 /2in slices 2 tablespoons vegetable oil 50g/2oz ricotta cheese, softened 2 tablespoons chopped fresh flat-leaf parsley 2 tablespoons chopped tomatoes salt and freshly ground black pepper

Preparation

• Brush the courgette slices with the oil, and grill on each side until lightly browned. Drain on kitchen paper and leave to cool.

• Mix the ricotta with the parsley, and season with salt and pepper. Spread this mixture on each courgette slice.

• Top each slice with some of the tomatoes and roll up, securing with a toothpick. Serve. 126 ingredients 225g/8oz Brie cheese 1 tablespoon chopped fresh flat-leaf parsley 1 tablespoon chopped sun-dried tomatoes in oil

• Preheat the oven to 230°C/ 450°F/Gas mark 8.

• Trim the rind from the top of the Brie, and place the Brie on a baking tray. In a small bowl, mix together the parsley and tomato.

• Spread the tomato mixture on top of the cheese, and bake in the oven for 10 minutes or until the cheese is heated through. Serve straight away.

Chive omelette stir-fry

ingredients

2 eggs 2 tablespoons snipped fresh chives 1 tablespoon groundnut oil 1 garlic clove, chopped 1cm/1 /2in piece of fresh root ginger, chopped 2 celery sticks, cut into shreds 2 carrots, cut into shreds 2 small courgettes, cut into shreds 1 bunch of radishes, sliced 4 spring onions, cut into shreds 100g/4oz beansprouts 1 /4 head Chinese leaves, shredded 1 tablespoon sesame oil salt and freshly ground black pepper

Preparation

• Whisk together the eggs and chives in a bowl. Season with salt and pepper, and whisk again. Heat about 1 teaspoon of the groundnut oil in a small frying pan, and pour in just enough of the egg mixture to cover the bottom of the pan. Cook for about 1 minute until set, then turn over and cook the omelette on the other side for a further minute.

• Tip out the omelette onto a plate, and cook the rest of the egg mixture in the same way to make two or three small omelettes, adding extra oil to the pan if necessary. Roll up each omelette and slice thinly. Keep the omelettes warm until required.

• Heat the remaining groundnut oil in a wok or large frying pan, add the garlic and ginger, and stir-fry for a few seconds.

• Add the celery, carrots and courgettes, and stir-fry for about 1 minute. Add the radishes, spring onions, beansprouts and Chinese leaves, and stir-fry for a further 3 minutes until all the vegetables are tender but still with a bite. Sprinkle the sesame oil over the vegetables, and toss gently.

• Serve the vegetables at once, with the omelette scattered over the top.

Egg curry

serves 4

ingredients

2 large onions, finely chopped 100g/4oz desiccated coconut 5 fresh red chillies 4 tablespoons tamarind

pulp 2 teaspoons coriander seeds pinch of asafoetida powder pinch of cumin seeds pinch of salt 2 eggs 2 tablespoons olive oil

Preparation

• To make the spice paste, put one-third of 1 onion in a large frying pan or wok over a medium heat with the coconut, chillies, tamarind, coriander seeds, asafoetida and cumin seeds. Toast for 5 minutes, stirring constantly. Remove from the heat and set aside to cool.

• Transfer the toasted spice mixture to a grinder, and grind for 2–3 minutes. Then, in a large heavy saucepan, combine the ground spices with the remaining two-thirds of 1 onion and 400ml/14fl oz water. Bring the mixture to the boil, reduce the heat and simmer for 5 minutes, stirring occasionally.

• Add the salt, then carefully break the eggs into the saucepan. Cover and cook for 5 minutes.

• In a frying pan, heat the oil, then add the remaining onion and cook over a high heat, stirring, until brown. Remove from the heat and pour the contents of the frying pan over the eggs. Serve hot.

French omelette

serves 2

ingredients

6 eggs 50g/2oz butter salt and freshly ground black pepper

Preparation

• Place a medium frying pan over a medium heat. Whisk the eggs in a bowl with salt and pepper until frothy. Put half the butter in the pan, tilting the pan to coat, then add half the eggs.

• Using the flat of a fork, stir the centre vigorously for 5 seconds, tilting the pan to move the uncooked egg to the edges. Remove from the pan while the middle is still slightly creamy, as the egg will continue cooking from residual heat. Repeat with the remaining butter and egg, and serve hot.

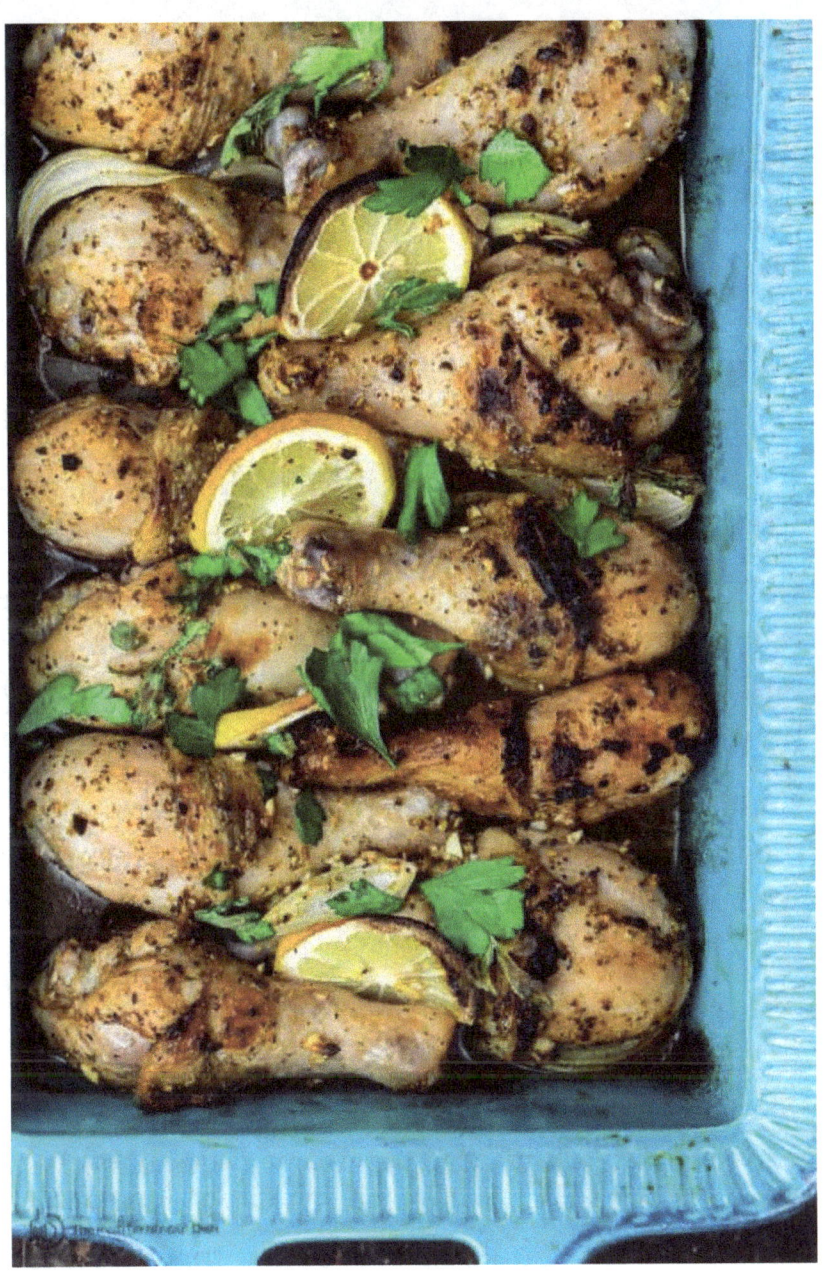

Pasta frittata

ingredients

350g/12oz spaghetti 4 eggs 1 /4 teaspoon ground black pepper 50g/2oz Parmesan cheese, freshly grated 2 tablespoons olive oil 100g/4oz mozzarella cheese, diced 2 tomatoes, diced 2 onions, chopped 50g/2oz prosciutto, sliced 2 tablespoons chopped fresh flat-leaf parsley

Preparation

• Add the spaghetti to a large saucepan of salted boiling water. Cook until al dente, drain, then cut into 2.5cm/1in lengths. Beat the eggs in a large bowl. Mix in the spaghetti, pepper and Parmesan.

• Heat the oil in a non-stick frying pan over a medium heat. Add half of the pasta mixture, spreading it out to the edges like a pancake. Spread the mozzarella in a single layer on top, then layer on the tomatoes, onions and prosciutto. Finish by spreading the remaining pasta on top and pouring any egg left in the bowl over it.

• Cook over a low heat for about 5 minutes. When the bottom has set and is golden brown, flip the frittata over. Cook, uncovered, for another 5 minutes or until the bottom is crisp and golden.

• To serve, cut into four wedges and sprinkle with parsley. Serve warm

Apple & Brie omelette

serves 4

ingredients

2 apples, peeled, cored and thinly sliced 25g/1oz butter 8 eggs 50ml/2fl oz single cream 100g/4oz Brie cheese, crumbled salt and freshly ground black pepper

Preparation

• Sauté the apple in half the butter over a medium heat. Beat together the eggs, cream and salt and pepper until blended but not frothy.

• Melt the remaining butter in a frying pan over a high heat until the foam begins to recede. Pour in the egg mixture. Cook the omelette, beating to lighten but allowing to set on the bottom. Fill with sautéed apples and Brie. Fold or roll, and slide out of the pan onto a heated plate.

Vegetable omelette

serves 6

ingredients

For the filling 25g/1oz butter 100g/4oz mushrooms, thinly sliced 1 courgette, cut into julienne 1 tomato, deseeded and coarsely chopped 1 /4 teaspoon salt 1 /8 teaspoon ground black pepper 2 tablespoons chopped fresh basil leaves 50g/2oz Parmesan cheese, grated For the omelette 12 eggs 1 tablespoon soda water 50g/2oz butter salt and freshly ground black pepper

Preparation

• To make the filling, heat the butter in a frying pan over a medium heat until melted. Add the mushrooms and sauté for 2 minutes. Add the courgette, and continue to sauté for 2 minutes.

• Add the tomato and cook over a high heat for 2 minutes to evaporate any excess liquid from the tomato. Add the salt, pepper and basil, and mix well. Taste for seasoning. Cover to keep warm.

• To prepare each omelette, whisk 2 eggs with a pinch of salt, a pinch of pepper and 1/2 teaspoon club soda until smooth.

• Melt 15g/1/2oz of the butter in a frying pan over a medium heat until it begins to sizzle.

• Pour in the egg mixture, and stir it in the centre of the pan with the flat side of a fork. Using the prongs of the fork, lift the edges of the omelette so pan. Vigorously slide the pan back and forth over the heat until the omelette begins to slip around freely.

• When the omelette is lightly cooked but still creamy in the centre, spoon about 2 tablespoons of the filling over the half of the omelette closer to the pan's handle. Sprinkle 1 tablespoon of the Parmesan over the filling.

• Fold the omelette in half, and slide the folded omelette onto a serving dish. Serve immediately. Repeat with the remaining eggs.

Indian eggs &chillies

ingredients

6 large eggs 3 tablespoons vegetable oil 4 green chillies, slit lengthways 2.5cm/1in piece of fresh root ginger, peeled and finely chopped 20 curry leaves 3 onions, finely sliced 3 tomatoes, sliced 1 /4 teaspoon ground turmeric 1 /4 teaspoon chilli powder pinch of salt

Preparation

• In a saucepan of water, slowly bring the eggs to the boil and simmer for 10 minutes until hard-boiled. Drain, remove the shells and set aside to cool.

• Heat the oil in a large pan and sauté the chillies, ginger and curry leaves for 2–3 minutes. Add the onions and fry until half-cooked.

• Add the tomatoes, turmeric, chilli powder and salt. Cook for 5 minutes or until thick. Add the whole eggs to the sauce, and mix gently until they are covered with the sauce. Remove from the heat, and serve hot with rice.

Piperade

serves 4

ingredients

1 onion, diced 75ml/3fl oz olive oil 3 red peppers, seeded and diced 11 /2 teaspoons red chilli flakes 4 ripe plum tomatoes, peeled and quartered 8 eggs salt and freshly ground black pepper

Preparation

• In a heavy pan over a low heat, sweat the onion in 3 tablespoons of the olive oil until soft and translucent.

• Add the peppers and chilli flakes. Continue to sweat over a low heat, stirring frequently, for 5–8 minutes.

• Add the tomatoes to the pan, season with salt and pepper, and cook until the mixture is thick and the tomatoes have broken down.

• Scramble the eggs in the remaining oil, seasoning to taste with salt and pepper. Fold the pepper purée into the eggs, and serve hot.

Spanish omelette

serves 4

ingredients

2 large potatoes, quartered 6 eggs 2 tablespoons olive oil 1 Spanish onion, chopped salt and freshly ground black pepper

Preparation

• Boil the potatoes in a saucepan of salted water for 15–20 minutes until just tender. Drain and leave until cool enough to handle, then cut the potatoes into slices.

• Beat the eggs in a bowl with salt and pepper to taste.

• Heat the oil in a deep non-stick frying pan over a low heat, add the onion and diced potatoes, and sauté for 10–15 minutes, stirring frequently, until soft and golden. Preheat the grill to hot.

• Add the eggs to the frying pan, and cook undisturbed for 5 minutes or until the eggs are just beginning to set in the centre. Slide the frying pan under the hot grill, and cook for a few minutes until the top is golden brown. Serve the omelette hot or cold, cut into wedges.

Pasta with caviar

serves 4

ingredients

225g/8oz fresh vermicelli 75g/3oz unsalted butter 100g/4oz good-quality caviar 8 fresh chives, chopped 8 quail's eggs, soft-boiled and peeled 1 lemon, thinly sliced

Preparation

• Cook the pasta in lightly salted boiling water until al dente, then drain, retaining a very little of the cooking water, and toss in the butter. Arrange in swirls on four small serving plates.

- Put a dollop of caviar in the centre of each mound of pasta, and sprinkle the chives over the top.

- Garnish each serving with two quail's eggs and lemon slices.

Spinach tagliatelle with veal

serves 4

ingredients

450g/1lb thin veal escalopes, cut into thin strips plain flour, seasoned 50g/2oz butter 1 onion, sliced 125ml/4fl oz dry white wine 4 tablespoons chicken stock 175ml/6fl oz double cream 600g/11 /4lb fresh spinach tagliatelle 3 tablespoons freshly grated Parmesan cheese salt and freshly ground black pepper

Preparation

- Dredge the veal strips with the seasoned flour. Melt the butter in a frying pan. Add the veal strips and sauté until browned. Remove with a slotted spoon, and set aside.

- Add the onion to the pan and sauté until soft and golden. Pour in the wine and cook rapidly to reduce the liquid. Add the stock and cream, and season with salt and pepper. Reduce the sauce again until it is thick and creamy, adding the veal towards the end.

• Meanwhile, cook the tagliatelle in a large pan of lightly salted boiling water until al dente. Drain and transfer to a warm serving dish.

• Stir 1 tablespoon of the Parmesan through the sauce, then pour the sauce over the pasta and toss gently to mix through. Serve immediately, sprinkled with the remaining Parmesan.

Pasta salad .

ingredients

450g/1lb penne 100g/4oz fresh basil leaves 2 garlic cloves, crushed 50g/2oz Parmesan cheese, freshly grated 2 tablespoons pine nuts, toasted 75ml/3fl oz olive oil 250g/9oz cherry tomatoes, halved 1 small red onion, sliced into thin wedges 150g/5oz pitted black olives

Preparation

• Cook the pasta in lightly salted boiling water until al dente. Drain, retaining a very little of the cooking water to keep moist. Set aside to cool while you make the pesto.

• Blend or process the basil, garlic, Parmesan and pine nuts until roughly chopped. With the motor running, add the oil in a thin stream until well combined.

• Put the pasta in a large bowl, stir in the pesto and mix well. Add the tomatoes, onion and olives. Stir gently. Chill for 1 hour, then serve

Pesto chicken salad

serves 4

ingredients

450g/1lb dried spiral pasta such as fusilli 125ml/4fl oz olive oil 2 tablespoons chopped pine nuts 2 tablespoons chopped fresh basil leaves 1 small onion, chopped 1 garlic clove, minced 900g/2lb skinless chicken thigh fillet, cubed 125ml/4fl oz red wine 1 tomato, diced 2 small carrots, chopped salt and freshly ground black pepper

Preparation

• Cook the pasta in lightly salted boiling water until al dente. Drain, retaining a little of the cooking water to keep moist. Cool while you make the rest of the salad.

• To make the dressing, mix the olive oil, pine nuts, basil, onion and garlic in a bowl. Season with salt and pepper. Refrigerate while you cook the chicken.

• Simmer the chicken cubes over a medium-high heat with 1 teaspoon salt and the red wine, stirring constantly, for about 10 minutes. When done, drain off the liquid.

• Toss together the chicken, dressing, tomato, carrots and pasta to serve. serves 6–8

Couscous salad

serves 2

ingredients

175g/6oz couscous 50g/2oz cooked peas Pinch of curry powder 2 spring onions (sliced) 1 small egg (hard-boiled and chopped) 2 tablespoons olive oil 2 teaspoons lemon juice Salt and pepper

Preparation

• Cook the couscous according to the packet instructions. Mix the couscous with the peas, curry powder, spring onions and egg.

• Toss with the olive oil and lemon juice, and season well with salt and pepper. Serve. 1

Rice salad

serves 6–8

ingredients

300g/11oz long-grain rice 75g/3oz frozen peas 3 spring onions, sliced 1 green pepper, finely diced 1 red pepper, finely diced 275g/10oz canned sweetcorn kernels, drained 15g/1 /2 oz fresh mint, chopped For the dressing 125ml/4fl oz extra virgin olive oil 2 tablespoons freshly squeezed lemon juice 1 garlic clove, crushed 1 teaspoon granulated sugar salt and freshly ground black pepper

Preparation

- Bring a large heavy pan of water to the boil, and stir in the rice. Return to the boil and cook for 12–15 minutes until tender. Drain and cool.

- Cook the peas in a small pan of boiling water for about 2 minutes. Rinse under cold water. Drain well.

- To make the dressing, whisk together the oil, juice, garlic and sugar in a small jug, then season with salt and pepper.

- Combine the rice, peas, spring onions, peppers, sweetcorn and mint in a large bowl.

- Pour over the dressing and mix well. Cover the salad with cling film, and refrigerate for 1 hour before serving.

Bean croquettes

ingredients

600g/11 /4lb canned cooked red kidney beans, drained 4 tablespoons butter 1 teaspoon vinegar 1 /4 teaspoon dried ground bay leaf 1 egg 12 tablespoons dried breadcrumbs vegetable oil for deep-frying salt and freshly ground black pepper

Preparation

- Blend the beans in a food processor until they form a smooth paste. Add the butter, vinegar and bay leaf. Season with salt and pepper. Blend for 2 minutes. Separate the mixture into 12 portions shaped like fingers.

• Beat the egg with some water, and put in a shallow dish. Put the breadcrumbs in another shallow dish.

• Coat the fingers, or croquettes, first with the egg, then with the breadcrumbs. Repeat the egg and breadcrumbs process to ensure that the croquettes are well coated. Chill for 1 hour.

• Heat enough oil for deep-frying in a heavy frying pan over a medium- high heat. When the oil is hot enough, deep-fry the croquettes until golden brown. Remove from the pan using a spatula or slotted spoon, and drain on kitchen paper. Serve hot.

Spinach & rice salad

serves 6-8

ingredients

225ml/8fl oz vinaigrette 1 teaspoon granulated sugar 300g/11oz cooked long-grain rice 200g/7oz fresh spinach, thinly sliced 100g/4oz celery, thinly sliced 150g/5oz spring onion, thinly sliced 100g/4oz streaky bacon, cooked and crumbled

Preparation

• Put the vinaigrette, soy sauce and sugar in a large salad bowl, and combine well. Add the rice and mix through well. Cover in cling film, and chill until ready to serve.

• Add the rest of the ingredients just before serving, and mix well. serves 6

Mixed bean salad

serves 4–6

ingredients

75g/3oz dried red kidney beans, soaked in cold water overnight 75g/3oz dried black-eyed beans, soaked in cold water overnight 75g/3oz dried borlotti beans, soaked in cold water overnight 125ml/4fl oz vinaigrette 1 tablespoon chopped fresh coriander leaves 1 onion, sliced into rings salt and freshly ground black pepper

Preparation

• Drain the kidney, black-eyed and borlotti beans. Put in a saucepan, cover with water and bring to the boil. Boil rapidly for 10 minutes, then simmer gently for 11 /2 hours until tender. Drain the cooked beans thoroughly, and put them in a large salad bowl.

• Combine the vinaigrette and coriander, and pour over the beans while they are still warm. Toss thoroughly and leave to cool for 30 minutes.

• Mix the onion into the beans, and season well with salt and pepper. Chill for 2–3 hours before serving. 138 Chickpea salad serves 6 ingredients 500g/1lb 2oz dried chickpeas, soaked in cold water overnight 2 large carrots 1 large onion 3 cloves garlic 4 tablespoons extra virgin olive oil 1 teaspoon salt 2 tablespoons white wine vinegar freshly ground black pepper

- Drain the beans and put in a saucepan. Cover with water and bring to the boil with the carrots, onion, garlic and 3 tablespoons of the olive oil. Simmer for 2 hours.

- Add the salt and simmer for a further hour until the chickpeas are cooked. Add water if necessary to keep them covered.

- Drain, reserving the liquid, but discarding the carrot, onion and garlic. Serve the chickpeas hot with a little of the liquid, a teaspoon of vinegar, the remaining olive oil and a sprinkling of pepper.

Rice-stuffed courgettes

. ingredients

4 courgettes, about 175g/6oz each 1 teaspoon sunflower oil 1 garlic clove, crushed 1 teaspoon ground lemon grass finely grated zest and juice of 1 /2 lemon 100g/4oz cooked long-grain rice 175g/6oz cherry tomatoes, halved 2 tablespoons cashew nuts, toasted salt and freshly ground black pepper

Preparation

- Preheat the oven to 200°C/400°F/Gas mark 6.

- Halve the courgettes lengthways, and use a teaspoon to scoop out the centres. Blanch the shells in boiling water for 1 minute, then drain well.

• Chop the courgette flesh finely, and put in a saucepan with the oil and garlic. Stir over a medium heat until softened but not browned.

• Stir in the lemon grass, lemon zest and juice, rice, tomatoes and cashew nuts. Season well with salt and pepper.

• Spoon the mixture into the courgette shells. Put the shells in a baking dish or roasting tin, and cover with foil. Bake for 25–30 minutes until the courgettes are tender

Lentil & rice salad

serves 6

ingredients

175g/6oz green lentils 200g/7oz basmati rice 4 large red onions, thinly sliced 4 garlic cloves, crushed 250ml/9fl oz olive oil 50g/2oz butter 2 teaspoons ground cinnamon 2 teaspoons sweet smoked paprika (pimentondulce) 2 teaspoons ground cumin 2 teaspoons ground coriander 2 spring onions, chopped salt and freshly ground black pepper

Preparation

• Cook the lentils and rice in separate pans of water until the grains are just tender, then drain.

• In a heavy pan over a low heat, very gently sweat the onions and garlic in the oil and butter for 30 minutes until very soft and caramelized. Stir in the cinnamon, paprika, cumin and coriander, and cook for a further 2 minutes until the spices are aromatic.

• Combine the onion and spice mixture with the drained rice and lentils. Stir in the spring onions, and season with salt and pepper. Serve warm.

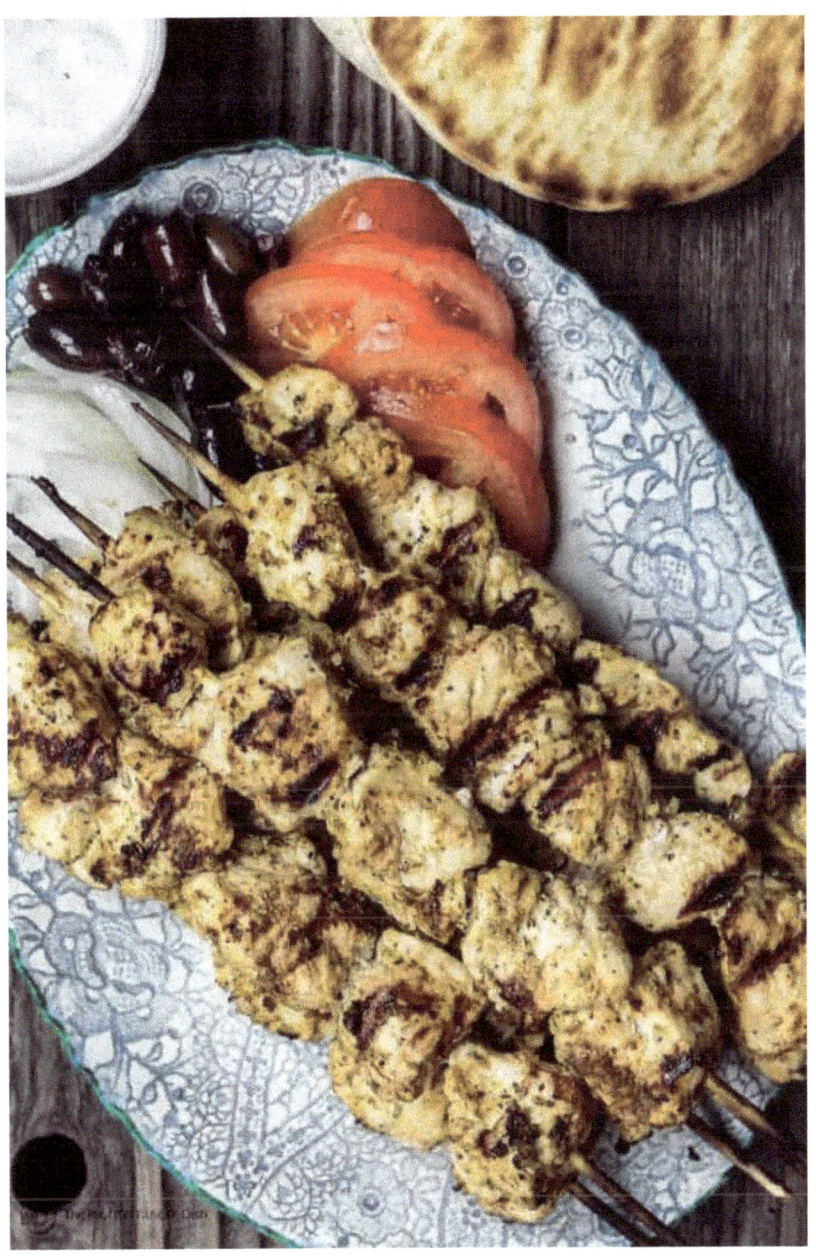

Spiced noodle salad

serves 4

ingredients

250g/9oz cooked rice noodles 175g/6oz broccoli, blanched 175g/6oz mangetout, blanched 2 teaspoons sesame oil 2 tablespoons plum sauce 4 tablespoons soy sauce 1 fresh red chilli, seeded and finely chopped

Preparation

• Mix the noodles with the broccoli and mangetout, and toss with the sesame oil, plum and soy sauces.

• Sprinkle with the chilli, and serve.

Stir-Fried Broccoli Pasta

ingredients

450g/1lb angel hair pasta 3 tablespoons olive oil 3 garlic cloves, finely chopped 1 head broccoli, broken into florets 2 red peppers, seeded and diced 250ml/9fl oz double cream 175g/6oz Parmesan cheese, freshly grated pinch of freshly grated nutmeg salt and ground black pepper

Preparation

• Cook the pasta in lightly salted boiling water for 8–10 minutes until just al dente. Drain, retaining just a little of the cooking water, then toss with 1 tablespoon of the oil. Keep warm.

• Heat the remaining oil in a heavy frying pan over a medium heat. Add the garlic and sauté lightly until soft (but do not brown). Add the broccoli and peppers, and sauté until tender.

• Remove the vegetables from the pan and set aside. Add the cream and bring to the boil. Reduce the heat and simmer for about 5 minutes until it starts to thicken. Add the Parmesan and a pinch of nutmeg, and cook for a further 2 minutes to thicken a bit more.

• Return the vegetables to the pan with the pasta, and toss together well. Season with salt and pepper if needed. Serve immediately.

1. Curried rice salad serves 6–8

ingredients

225ml/8fl oz vinaigrette 1 tablespoon curry powder 1/2 teaspoon salt 250g/9oz cold cooked long-grain rice 6 scallions, chopped 4 celery sticks, finely chopped 2 red peppers, seeded and finely chopped

Preparation

• In a small bowl, whisk together the vinaigrette, curry powder and salt to make the dressing.

• Put the remaining ingredients in a medium bowl. Add the dressing, and toss until combined.

• Cover with cling film, and chill for at least 2 hours before serving.

Mushroom Risotto

serves 4

ingredients

1 onion, finely chopped 2 tablespoons olive oil 450g/1lb portobello mushrooms, stalks removed if woody, halved and thickly sliced 350g/12oz risotto rice such as Arborio or Carnaroli 150ml/5fl oz dry white wine 1 litre/13 /4pt hot vegetable stock 25g/1oz butter 3 tablespoons freshly grated Parmesan cheese

Preparation

• In a large heavy saucepan over a gentle heat, sweat the onion in the olive oil for about 15 minutes unti soft and caramelized.

• Increase the heat and add the mushrooms, sautéeing for 3–4 minutes until browned. Add the rice and cook, stirring, for a further minute until the grains are coated in oil.

• Pour in the white wine and simmer, stirring constantly, until the liquid has been almost completely absorbed.

• Meanwhile, keep a pan of the vegetable stock simmering on the stove. Add a ladleful of vegetable stock to the rice. Simmer, stirring, until the liquid has been absorbed. Continue adding the stock in this way, stirring continuously, until all the stock has been used and the rice is tender.

• Remove from the heat, stir in the butter and Parmesan, and serve hot.

Fresh herb risotto

ingredients

1 tablespoon olive oil 1 onion, finely chopped 2 garlic cloves, finely chopped 225g/8oz risotto rice such as Arborio or Carnaroli 215ml/4fl oz dry white wine 700ml/11 /4pt hot vegetable stock 3 tablespoons chopped fresh mixed herbs such as basil, parsley, chives and chervil finely grated zest of 1 lemon salt and ground black pepper Parmesan cheese shavings, to serve

Preparation

• Heat the oil in a medium heavy pan over a low heat. Gently sweat the onion and garlic until soft and starting to caramelize.

• Add the rice, and cook, stirring, over a low to medium heat for 1–2 minutes until all the grains are coated in oil.

• Pour in the white wine and simmer, stirring constantly, until the liquid has been almost completely absorbed.

• Meanwhile, keep a pan of the stock simmering on the stove. Add a ladleful of stock to the rice. Simmer, stirring, until the liquid has been absorbed. Continue adding the stock in this way, stirring, until all the stock has been used and the rice is tender.

• Remove from the heat, stir in 2 tablespoons of the herbs and the lemon zest. Season well with salt and pepper. Serve hot, garnished with the remaining herbs and Parmesan shavings.

Spaghetti with garlic &chilli oil

serves 2

ingredients

250g/9oz dried spaghetti 75ml/3fl oz extra virgin olive oil 4 garlic cloves, crushed 1 small fresh red chilli, seeded and finely chopped 6 tablespoons chopped fresh flat-leaf parsley

• Cook the pasta in a large pan of salted boiling water until al dente.

• Meanwhile, heat the olive oil over a gentle heat, and sauté the garlic and chilli for about 3 minutes until the garlic turns lightly golden.

• Remove from the heat and pour over the drained cooked pasta, and mix in the parsley. Serve hot.

Seafood spaghetti

serves 4

ingredients

350g/12oz dried spaghetti 500g/1lb 2oz mussels 700g/11 /2lb squid, cleaned 500g/1lb small littleneck clams 300g/11oz shrimps 4 cloves garlic 6 tablespoons extra virgin olive oil 250ml/9fl oz dry white wine 3 tablespoons chopped fresh flat-leaf parsley 2 dried red chillies, finely chopped salt and freshly ground black pepper

Preparation

• Soak the mussels and clams in water for an hour. Discard any broken mussels or clams, or open ones that don't close when tapped on the work surface. Under cold running water, scrub the mussels and clams thoroughly to remove any grit, pulling out the beards from the mussels.

• In a large deep frying pan over a medium heat, sweat 1 clove of the garlic in 2 tablespoons of the oil. Increase the heat to high, and add the mussels and clams with half of the wine. Cover with a tight-fitting lid, and cook for about 5 minutes until the shells are open (discard any that remain closed). Remove from the heat and discard the garlic.

• Slice the squid into rings and finely chop the remaining garlic. Heat the remaining oil in another pan, and sauté the garlic, parsley and chillies for a few minutes. Add the squid and cook until the edges curl.

• Pour in the remaining wine and cover. Cook for 10 minutes. Add the shrimps (just the tails) and cook for a few more minutes before adding the clams and mussels. Simmer for another few minutes, then remove from the heat.

• Meanwhile, bring a large saucepan of salted water to the boil, add the spaghetti and cook until al dente. Drain and add the seafood mixture to the spaghetti, mixing well.Stir over a low heat for a couple of minutes. Serve piping hot

Cheese-Stuffed Rice Balls

ingredients

200g/7oz long-grain rice, cooked and cooled 2 eggs, lightly beaten 100g/4oz mozzarella cheese, cubed 100g/4oz coarse dried breadcrumbs vegetable oil for deep-frying

Preparation

• Mix together the rice and egg until well combined. Take a teaspoon of the rice and put a mozzarella cube in the centre. Top with another teaspoon of rice. Press together to form a ball. Continue until all the rice mixture has been used.

• Coat the rice balls with the breadcrumbs. Place on a baking tray, and refrigerate for at least 30 minutes. Heat enough oil for deep-frying in a heavy pan. Fry the rice balls, in batches, for 5 minutes until golden brown. Serve hot.

Broad Bean, Pea & Goat's Cheese Salad

serves 4

ingredients

250g/9oz goat's cheese 1 bunch of watercress leaves 1 tablespoon chopped fresh tarragon 1 tablespoon chopped fresh flat-leaf parsley 2 spring onions, finely sliced 75g/3oz peas 100g/4oz broad beans, skinned 4 tablespoons olive oil 1 tablespoon lemon juice 1 tablespoon freshly grated Parmesan cheese salt and ground black pepper

Preparation

• Preheat the grill until hot. Cut the goat's into thick slices, and season with salt and pepper. Cook under the grill for 3–4 minutes until the cheese starts to melt.

• Toss the herbs with the spring onions, peas, broad beans, oil, lemon juice and Parmesan. Season with salt and pepper.

• Top the salad with the goat's cheese, and serve straight away.

Chinese Lettuce Wraps

serves 4

ingredients

450g/1lb minced beef 12–16 iceberg lettuce leaves 225g/8oz canned water chestnuts, drained and chopped 200g/7oz onion, chopped 2 tablespoons minced garlic 2 tablespoons light soy sauce 50ml/2fl oz hoisin sauce 2 teaspoons minced fresh root ginger 1 tablespoon rice wine vinegar 1 tablespoon chilli sauce 1 bunch of spring onions, chopped 3 teaspoons dark sesame oil

Preparation

• Sauté the beef and onion in a large frying pan over a medium heat. Add the garlic, soy sauce, hoisin sauce, ginger, vinegar and chilli sauce. Continue stirring and cooking until browned.

• Add the water chestnuts, spring onions and sesame oil. Stir and cook for a further 1–2 minutes.

• To serve, arrange the lettuce leaves on the outer rim of a large serving plate. Put the meat mixture in the centre of the plate. To eat, spoon the meat mixture on the lettuce and wrap the leaf around the filling.

CPSIA information can be obtained
at www.ICGtesting.com
Printed in the USA
LVHW081817240321
682333LV00003B/109